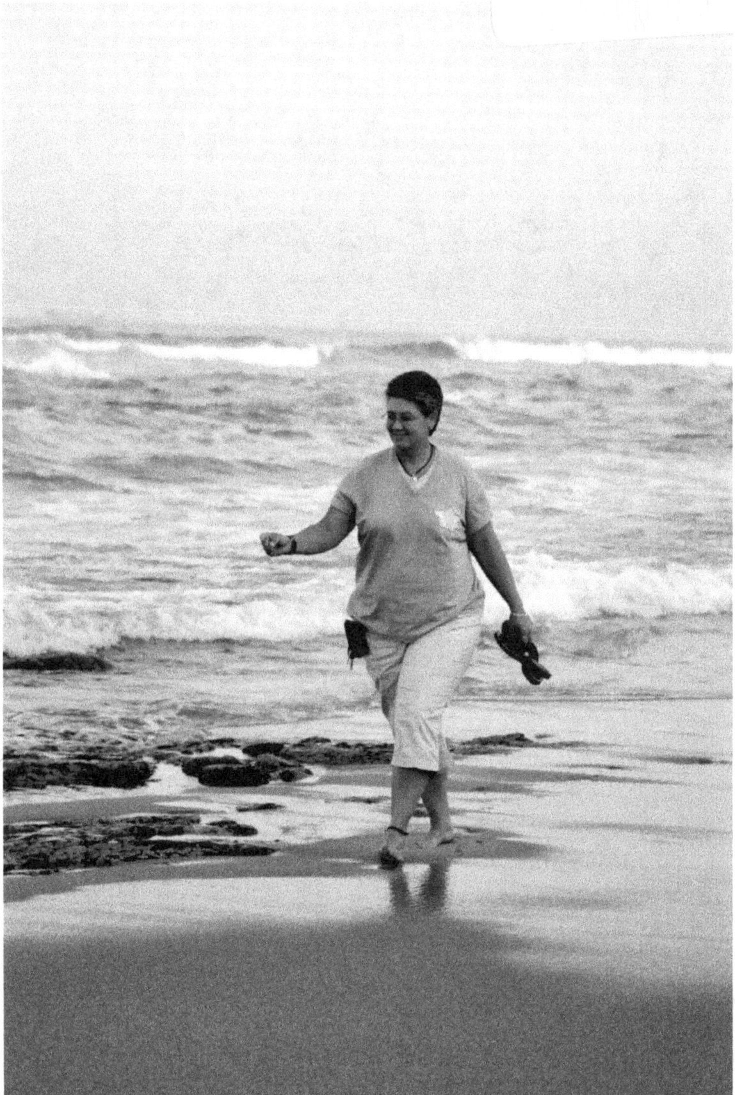

Endit Eating Plan

Behind the food

You will never touch another diet after you read this.

Written by

Chris Gillam

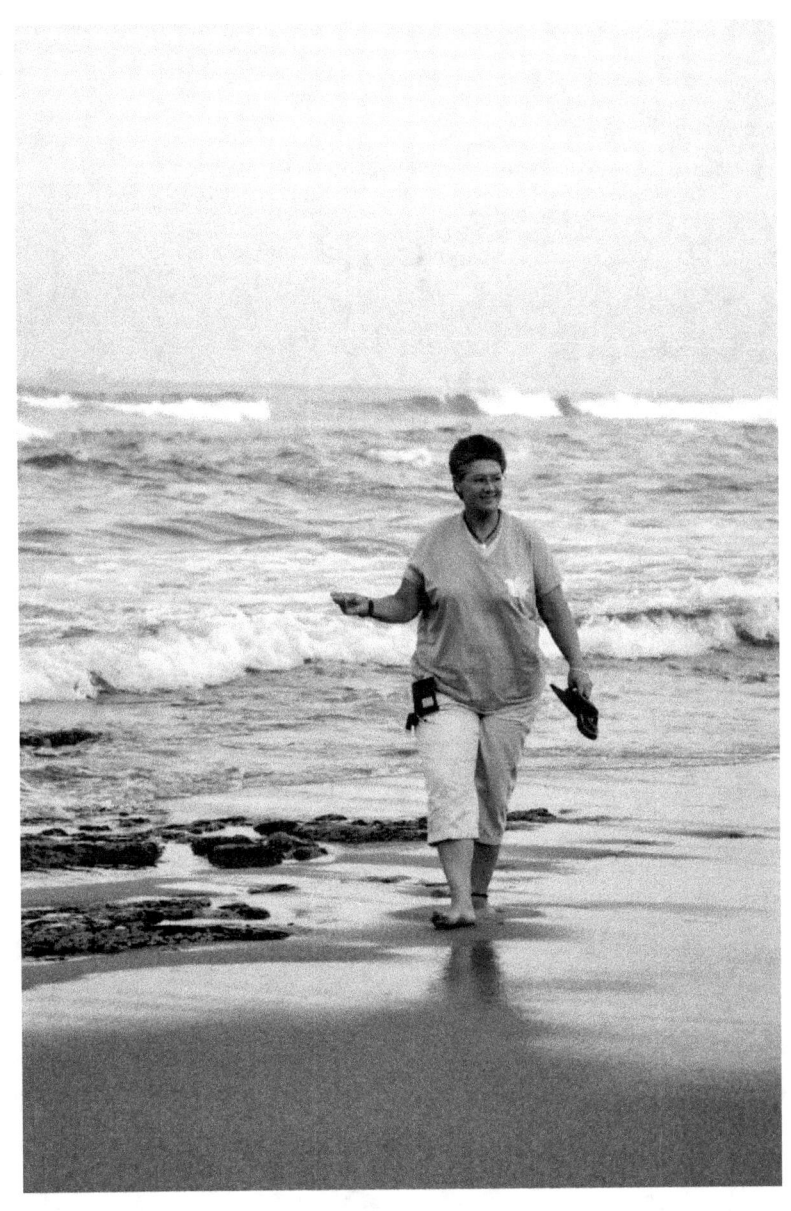

Credits

Edited by
Susan Ames

Hairdressing
Val Murray

Dietician
Dr. Carol Potgieter

Cover Designer
Adam Saviddes

Published by Writersink 20/10/2014

Contents

Writersink ™ RSA

Athlone Park

Durban

Kwa-Zulu Natal

Phone 27.31.904.1260

Hardcopy

Printed by BK Bookbinders

Durban North

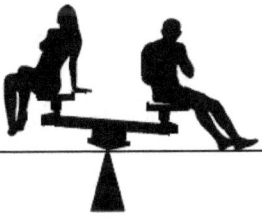

The ENDIT way

Understand your relationship with food

There are literally millions of diet books, diet plans and diet products available and the biggest and most successful ones are the American diets which are written mainly for the Hollywood and Californian regions but publicity houses send them across the globe and Jane and Joe Average buy into the plan or rather fund the huge commercial daisy chain of diet and weight reduction commerce.

A small fact that many average people overlook is that we are not Hollywood stars, we are Mr, Mrs and Miss Average. We do not live in a world of beauty and self absorption. We have to go to work, earn a living, pay bills and look after our families and our kids all of which take 110% of our time and resources.

Those diets are for single people and the commitment you need to them is insane. I have personally tried a large number of them all.

I was diagnosed as being clinically obese 5 years ago and strangely I have never had a great relationship with food. I do not like a lot of food on my plate. I do not like mushy food. I was never a big eater; I am a picky eater, I like something today and off it tomorrow, I have an amazing sense of smell and anything with the slightest offensive odour and I wont touch it, I can smell the table surface at a restaurant and if it has the slightest "lap" smell I leave and I am a Type 1 diabetic. I was not a snacks type person, I always liked fruit and I was never a drinker. I don't like take away food or Chinese take away, to me beef is not grey pink when cooked so maybe it is a derivative of beef of another kind.

My weight was fine, manageable and like anyone always thought a few kilograms lost would do no harm and suddenly I began packing on the kilo's. I ballooned. Nothing fitted, waistline became wasteland, face neck and shoulders became one and the same, upper arms hung like satchels, hip bones long lost, my thighs chaffed and inner seams of pants wore to holes. My weight ballooned from 75kg to 147kg.

(In pounds that is 323). My height being 5ft7. That is a whole human being of extra weight. My pants size went from a size 36 to a mans size 46 and they were still tight and straining. My trousers on a washing line, pegging it on one side of the waist band to the other took up ½ of the length of line. I hung my clothing out to dry at night, too ashamed of the neighbours seeing my clothing. One of my thighs looked like the entire middle trunk of a person and my size five feet looked like they were a size 3, encased in a bulge of fat.

I was a person lost in a body of blubber.

Fat was not only killing me it was also killing my budget. I collapsed one bed, then another. The third one the plastic foot broke off on my side of the bed, by then I could not afford another bed so we took all the feet off the bed.

Shame and depression set in, avoiding friends and family, occasions and events were normal now. I had nothing to wear anyway. Doctors prescribed antidepressants and sleeping pills. I was suicidal. I was depressed for good reason and was not sleeping because I was depressed and worried and the worst possible thing a depressed person can do for themselves is take to bed.

I gave up on food. My logic was if it is not in the body it cannot grow any fatter, at some point the body would have to start using itself and I would loose the weight again. Not so. The body is not made to feed on itself no matter what stories you read. Unless you physically bite pieces of yourself off and eat it, the body is not going to eat itself. It will use energy but energy is not the same as fat reserves and starving yourself damages many other organs including skin, hair, nails, liver, kidneys, brain, central nervous system, eyes and teeth and starving yourself and trying to work, just don't do it. Your memory and balance are also impaired much like trying to drive after a couple of pain killers. Yes it is possible, but safely, not so. Your judgement is off and your boss will notice. Simply put it is like trying to make a car run on petrol fumes.

I hated myself, I was filled with disgust and fat rolls, I stopped looking at myself in any mirror. I entered the world of diets and the cycle of self abuse, self degradation and contempt. In this self hatred you are also bordering on mental illness as you demean yourself and punish yourself as if you were two separate entities.

I began with the soup diet, hmmm that one. You remember it do you? The cabbage, onions and green peppers. I got through two pots of it.

Today if I eat cabbage once a year it is a lot. Then I did the laxatives and orange juice diet. All I achieved was a stomach ulcer. That is possibly the most painful thing you could do to yourself. The expenses involved to fix it are more than you want to incur and unless you enjoy constant pain that feels like a stab wound in your gut, this is not the way to go about it. This pain drains you. It wakes you up, it prevents sleep, it makes you irritable and you cannot eat much with this pain but you have to eat because you stomach produces acids which worsen it and even if you walk past food it stimulates acids. You are sick all the time. It takes long to heal.

Then I moved into the big leagues, the American diets. With the one, the teeth in my mouth loosened due to the over consumption of protein. At first I thought it was sensitivity. I tried the various and expensive toothpastes. They did not help. I went to the dentist. My teeth were loose, all of them. You could move them with your finger which allowed nerve exposure. She told me that if it became worse I would lose them all. I would need plates. I had lost some weight but nothing close to what it promised and between the diet food and the dentist, it was not worth it at all.

The other with the over consumption of acid food like strawberries, watermelon and citrus, my hair began to fall out and I had perpetual thrush. Thrush is very uncomfortable and it also smells bad.

Now if we were in Hollywood or California or the places where all the exceptionally beautiful people live with surgeons as common as garden services, then we could go have a new set of teeth implanted and new hair sewn into our scalps...but sadly for us, our reality is family, kids, car pools, jobs and weight .

My reality kicked in when I collapsed in a parking lot late in the evening with my car door open, my wallet and phone on the seat and keys in hand. I was about to get into the car after buying more spinach and soda water. I was admitted to the closest hospital by strangers. Kind and honest strangers as all my belongings were in tact. My younger sister came to the hospital with a psychologist friend of hers. I was not only in physical trouble, I was in mental trouble and I was unhappy. That sad unhappiness that sits like a wet sheet over you for no apparent reason other than it just is. The sun shines unseen, the rain falls unseen, life is a blur of automated action. That kind of hopeless unhappiness.

With a few sessions with the psychologist of venting my anger and frustration at the condition of my body, the whys and the wherefores I actually felt better. Just getting it out there, identifying it, naming and shaming it, telling someone I was fat and angry and did not want this body as it was like a fine intelligent engine with a whale of dead meat around me and people looked at me differently, that pitiful expression in their eyes, that fat person tolerance, the nervous look when I went to sit on a chair, would the legs break or the wheels crack off look and the relief when it held.

I changed doctors and I educated myself on the workings of the human body in consultation with several dieticians. It so turned out my insulin doses were totally incorrect and in conflict with other conditions I had. The diagnosis was a relief and the medications changed however I was still stuck with dilemma of the walking mini bus sized body. Changing medication is like signing a treaty of peace, the problem lies in the fact that the live landmine does not know it is now at peace. It would be weeks before the new medications turned the process around and that would just mean I would not continue gaining weight but it did not mean it would reverse what had already happened or automatically reduce me back to my original size and magically all my wardrobe would fit. With the morbid obesity came a heart condition, water retention, sleep aponia, bronchitis, and blood pressure problems over and above constant back ache.

I took my life, my eating, my medications, my health and my attitude into my own control. I was done with the books and the shakes, drops, magic pills, teas, scales and every thing that had the word "slim" was binned and trashed. One sentence that was said to me by a dietician was the magic phrase after spending tens of thousands.

"If nature made it you can eat it, and always eat only sufficient for your need".

We all have a chemical in our brain that triggers in when we are sufficiently full, and it cuts off your need to eat further. Recognise the signals. Make your food presentable, enjoy it, have fun with it. You deserve to eat and eat well but eat right. Eat don't feed.

Make that platter for a Saturday afternoon when friends visit or make it for yourself when you are chilling and camping in front of the TV or in the garden, fill it with light snack biscuits and fresh vegetables and fruits, a healthy dip and snack away. It is snacking but it is not sausage rolls and pastry, it is not chips and burgers.

No different than filling your car up with petrol and throwing a can of oil in behind it into the petrol tank. The car is going to die.

I have lost 71kg in total. I do not have pockets of hanging skin that requires any surgery at all. I am not flabby. No miracle and minimal exercise as well. I am not inactive but I am not a gym buff either. I do not run around the blocks, I don't even own running shoes. I walk like you do. Around the stores, in the malls, in the parking, nothing astronomical. I will park far from the entrance, more to preserve my car doors but it does give you a little more walking exercise, if you tend to have back ache, don't be discouraged from walking the entire length of the mall, just use a trolley to hold onto as support, you will not lie on the trolley for long as they are really uncomfortable on your arms so you will find the way to walk just holding the handles for support, but you are still walking. When you walk, be conscious of walking, don't slop alone, move your legs in the manner they should be used, forward keeping your back straight. Use your hips, if you push them slightly forward you will be less inclined to step side to side like your one leg is shorter than the other. Take the lift, use the escalator, enjoy being everywhere around the mall. The concept of "take the stairs only" …well yeah…I suppose there is a place for people in the world with all that going on in them too. We are not them. I have found as I developed more mobility and began to enjoy my own body I have looked for exercises to do and enjoy being active. I swim more, I now do own gym equipment and I have developed the illusive 6 pack stomach. I now fit a size 36/37 pants, have to wear a belt and do not enjoy wearing too lose or too big clothing and I certainly, even with a trim body do not like over tight clothing either. Realise that this body is you and make friends with it. Your body, your mind, your soul and your smile…they are all one. They all make up the wonderful YOU. Don't' hurt it, don't abuse it and always respect it. We always believe for some strange reason that we will go on, no matter what. Well I realised that my body is the house for my soul and when that body stops and dies, my soul leaves, gone and the people that love me and depend on me, well they will go on, but with a hole that I would have created in their lives.

If you lose weight too fast you will have the pocket of skin hanging from your stomach, your body needs to adjust all the time and as you lose so will your body adjust as will your mobility increases. Light stretching, carpet stretching, swing ball, hand ball, swimming if you have access to a pool, gardening, carrying your groceries one bag at a time into your house forces you to walk up and down, bending to pat your pets, stretching to close curtains from the rail, these are all things that you make part of your existence, take the time, enjoy the movement and know that your body is gaining more life, more blood flow, more metabolism with each movement. Increase your exercise and do more as you can and you will find a new lease on life. Massage, if you can afford it, I highly recommend it. Tone your body, do everything to avoid the pockets of drooping skin. Keep blood flow and energy all through the body. Don't watch pockets of flesh forming. It is your body, manage it. The surgery is expensive and very invasive and yes you can hide the tummy scar but not so easy to hide the zip scars on your legs that will go from your ankle to your groin and not always do we heal well. The scar could be light or it could be a thick ugly inch wide skew pink crevice. Rather do it the hard way now as in the end it will be the easier way and healthier way.

Plastic surgery can cost from R80 000 to R600 000, depending on corrective procedures and complications.

There is no need to go sign up with the gym, buy exercise equipment, cycles, join running groups. Walk at your pace, stop and see the view, watch people, take the rest break on the bench. You and your body are re-building their relationship. Don't fight it, don't hate it and don't hurt it. I made myself a rope exerciser. Clearly by my weight you could see I was not going to a gym, I could not run (could barely walk without having to sit down to rest) and this allowed me to use my arms to lift my legs, so it was natural resistance using my own body weight. It also allowed me to gain suppleness and lower back and core strength. It burnt calories and I would put my head phones on and just go at my own pace. It was my time out in my space without intrusion or eyes.

In my weight loss journey I did not starve myself. I have eaten cake and chocolates, crisps, burgers, ribs, baked potato, lamb, braai, pap…. I have not taken any drugs, I have not used any formulation, drops, shakes or anything of the like. I paid tens of thousands for what I will share with you. I learnt invaluable knowledge. I travelled thousands of kilometres to various specialists. 71kg of weight loss is no small feat. Think about 71 blocks of butter packed onto your back, legs, arms, butt, hips chest and stomach.

We will cover the products you have or are taking.

We will cover the psychology of a weighted person.

We will cover choices vs. decisions.

Past and present.

Feel good and emotion

Dressing properly and stylish options and alternatives which will include photos and pics will be included in the online program for you to use at will, take from them, experiment and bring out your best features.

No eating plan formulated allows you to check off your desired foods for the day and calculates your calories. You formulate what you want to eat.

It includes recipes and tips of optimising your food

Oprah's battle with binge eating

You will be linked in to your plan which is interactive. You can leave notes, hints, tips and your own discoveries for others.

It is perfect for children, men, teens and older seniors.

No fancy food that you need to break the budget to buy.

No special purchases. No brand names punted.

Work with what you have in the kitchen.

Take control of your decisions.

No Monthly subscriptions. On sell and intro to others if you see the benefit of it which I know you will and actually earn while you loose. We pay R24.99 per copy sold and how you market or who you market to is yours. It is in the on sales that prevents people pirating copy for give away's. The cost of the sales goes into the development of the programming for you. Respect the plan as it is yours as if you had created it for yourself. Our software does allow us to track unauthorised log in activity and we can track it back to origination and we will delete the pirate as well as the origin log in with no refund.

Become an ambassador and earn real money, not discounts, stars or points.

Super fast always accessible engine available for you even on your smartphone.

Fluid information constantly updating

Become part of a community and have support from many without criticism as we only advocate support, kindness and generosity of spirit.

No weighing in. Be your guide. Be comfortable in yourself.

Go steady and go slow, if you lose too fast you will see the benefit of the loss of weight and inches but seriously, you do not want the pockets of skin hanging around your knees.

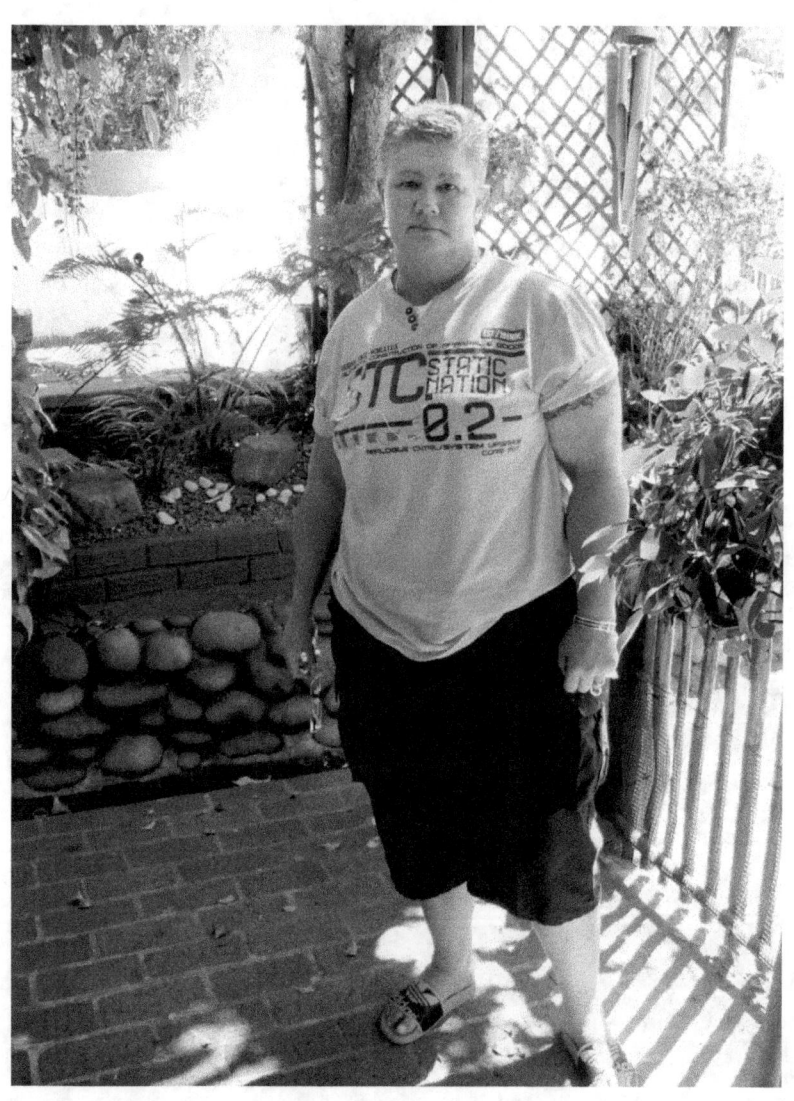

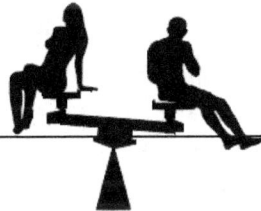

Diet Products

There are very few I have not tried or seen tried by friends and family.

Look at the cost of them...nothing cheap about them for what you are getting.

Now look at the logic...Every single one of them is a con and a scam. There is no such thing as burning off 4kg in 5 days because you did not even put 4kg of weight onto your body in 5 days. If you were able to pack on 4kg of weight in 5 days you would be incapable of movement at all, you would be a huge blob of flesh. The body cannot process like that and neither can it do it in reverse. You can lose the weight in the same time you packed it on if you just changed your eating habits. So if you packed on 20 kilos of weight over a year period, you can lose it again over a year with minimal effort.

But we always want the good stuff in a hurry. We want instant weight loss and products promise us these wonderful results and then they have testimonials of woman and men standing with the before and after photos and none of us look too closely at them. They are similar but it is not the same person at all and where replication and similarity fails photo editing takes over.

Logically and biologically, we have been lazy, inactive, eaten the fatty nice things and sat in sloth mode for months, years and lifetimes and we expect a couple of drops of "all natural" tincture in a glass of water to dissolve away the fat and give us the toned supple body of someone who spends hours refining muscle and eating greens to do. Now analyse the marketing, really take notice of the marketing. She stands under photographic lighting, placed strategically in a setting of optimal performance after hours of professional makeup to tell you she has lost 7kg in 10 days, 2 weeks, etc but here is the closer…."and I have never felt better", "I am happier than I have ever been", "I got my life back", "I feel more energetic" or the visual aids…"she is running with her child on the beach towards a good looking perceptively well to do man wearing wither khaki or baby blue or white clothing".

Lets look at the verbiage first…."I am happier than I have ever been", this translates in your mind to "I can be happy". "I have never felt better", this translates in your mind to "I can feel better", "I got my life back" (These are the most powerful words in marketing, used in advertising of dental glue to adult nappies) and translates in your mind to a time when you felt happier and can regain that period.

Diet products are the most successfully sold products across the globe second only to cosmetic wrinkle creams and skin whitening and lightening products and are targeted mainly at woman for a simple reason. Woman are emotional. The base workings of a woman's brain is driven primarily on emotive purchasing. Not whim purchases, that is another study entirely. This is emotive in the purest form.

Sex appeal, acceptance, self esteem, attractiveness to others, envy, ego are all linked to our rush to buy instant reform products.

When we were 18 years old even though we did not recognise it in ourselves at the time and always aspired to be the "in" crowd, the jock or the popular girl and we felt gawky and awkward in ourselves we realised later that that time was actually a happy time, we were safe in our lives then, parents, grandparents, aunts and uncles, family time and closeness.

We moved on to dating and it was fun, we were thin and pretty or handsome, we looked good, we were trim and lean and of course we were always careful about what we ate, seriously who was going to be seen wolfing down a double cheese, chips and shake? Friends were our natural guide of "you don't want to be seen eating that" and even though we hung out in those pizza places, how much did you really eat and how much did you share. I well remember one pizza and upward 5 hands reaching for a slice. Life was about careless whispers and potential marriages, the first child and our whole futures were in front of us.

Then life took over.

Jobs, bonds, bills, debt, divorce, 2nd marriage, maintenance fights, teenagers and we were suddenly our parents. Working all day and coming home to cook, homework, making lunch and husbands/wives, life planning, bickering and we became less and less important to ourselves. Healthy food became "economical" food, meal planning became "warm ups" with a few slices of bread, Ice creams with a romantic date became comfort food and taking care of ourselves became consolation foods.

We made these choices and then we expected our bodies to fit in with them and into the sizes we once fitted.

We tell ourselves things so that we do not have to put in the effort. A chest pain is not always the reflux of eating on the run, it sometimes is plain and simply a warning signal but even that is fobbed off to "stress or a carbonated drink" when we should really see a doctor but in the back of our minds we already know what they are going to say, diet and exercise and those are the two last things we want addressed as it may interrupt our lives, for as long as we will still have the privilege of them.

Have you ever looked at your dinner table and taken you mind back to when you were a kid? When did your mom ever serve macaroni cheese with sausages and basket of rolls and a 2 litre cola?

When were we ever allowed to eat endless burgers and pizza slices?

Those were not dinner table foods, those were for parties. Those were pretty rare too.

We now serve that as a dinner meal and wonder why our kids are over weight, inflamed with acne and have social issues and eating disorders.

We go and drive and spend time in a queue to get the burger with fries and cola and a chocolate bar or ice creams thrown in for free and we feed our families these poisons and expect them to achieve and stay healthy. This is insanity. Grease, fat, sugar and colorants are not food and they are not cheap either.

Choices we make and made and our parents and grandparents sit in shock and horror shaking their heads and we console ourselves with the phrase, "the world is a different place now". But our bodies don't know that, we have not evolved that fast, as fast as a computer can come up with another chemical or colour or flavour.

Our bodies still need the same nutrition people did 200 years ago to function well and effectively.

We see the attractive woman running on the beach with her 5 year old towards the man of her dreams in the advert, she is slim and healthy and has the hair blowing in the wind, and she is the middle aged perfection of wife version of Baywatch. The perfect family but it is not your family. He is a model, as is she and the kid.

You look around and you have the sullen teen with the acne and the irritable over fed bloating husband manning the remote control, while your pizza slices are warming in the oven with the diet soda on the table and your mind says to you...

"I need to buy that, I need to be happy, I need to get my life back" and it is not the product that is selling itself to you, it is the lifestyle behind the product.

The product could be tap water in a dark brown bottle with a dropper attached and a fancy label. You do not care if it works or not, you are already in the grip of diet products, you know before you buy it that it is not going to work, but you will happily use it for maybe a week at a stretch, you will continue to eat pizza slices for dinner and burgers for lunch and put your 5 drops of whatever into your glass of water and think your whole miserable self will change, all because of a few drops of who knows what from a bottle?

You are not looking for a product; you are really looking for a remedy to your life.

Diet products come in all forms, from shakes in tins to drops, from powders to injections. They do not work. When you are totally devoted for the first couple of days, you lose a bit, mostly water as every single diet plan comes with the same universal instruction, drink 4 – 8 glasses of water per day. If you did that and continued to eat as you are, you would still lose some weight as you will still process your metabolism better with water, use the bathroom more, evacuate your bowl more frequently and you have changed nothing but drank more water. I have known a number of people who have had the "injections". They really do work. No they honestly do. One friend of mine lost 33kg in 9 months. However, there are two types of injections. Neither of which is actually any "diet" miracle. One has a completely normal over the counter mineral of relatively high dosage and the injections cost you anything upward R2500 for a 6 week course accompanied by a very strict meal planner and the other type of injection is pure vitamin B12 which burns like fire and are very painful and accompanied by a very rigid strict eating plan which will set you back R3000 for the 6 weeks. The first is a supplement with a diet plan, the second is a immunity enhancer with a diet plan.

When you stop either program you balloon, back to your old size plus half. The supplement causes your digestive system to race so you process food faster and it passes faster, the second is a booster so you feel good and energetic like you are on a feel good high, not spaced out high, just really good.

My friend was almost suicidal and actually has never lost the weight, basically gave up, lived with it and has not even lost the extra added bonus kilos. No one can remain on those shots for 52 weeks of the year unless you have R30 000 a year to inject plus doctors consult fees as they do add those on even if it is reduced rates and medical aids do not cover the shots either.

Realistically that is a full and comprehensive grocery budget for one person per month or a child's school fees per month, a very good contribution to a retirement plan.

So when these advertisers market these products they are using years and years and billions of cash value in research to hit at your most urgent and screaming out last nerve even if that nerve is buried deep within fat. They reach it and you reach into your last cash reserves in the hope of obtaining the miracle of you.

Never buy into "doctor approved" or "developed by a doctor" formulation of a diet product. No *medical* doctor would dismiss all your life into a bottle of drops. No *medical* doctor would advocate the use of drugs that put you on a high and accelerate your heart rate, place you on a protein only or fruit only diet. When you see "doctor approved" it could be anyone with a doctorate, in music, in philosophy, but not a *medical* doctor.

Diet products are commercial gain value only, and it is sad that woman from as early as the 1950's began on this perpetual wheel of weight loss. I am old enough to remember when woman were taking tablets that contained a tapeworm eggs so that the worms could hatch in their stomachs and they would literally cause themselves to be starved by an intestinal parasites as long as they lost weight and were stick thin. The statement made by Wallace Simpson of you can never bee "too rich or too thin".

Today being stick thin means a lot of other unattractive things to us. Alcoholism, eating disorders, bulimia, HIV and poverty but in that none of us wants to be overweight or fat either.

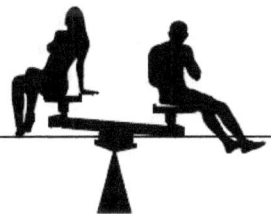

Diet clubs and clinics

Dieting is like dating, always to do it better with a friend or a few friends.

When you have issues, good or bad issues with your husband, wife, lover, girlfriend, boyfriend, new person of interest, you call someone, your mate, your best girl, sister, mom or at worst discuss with a co-worker but always better with a friend. Well dieting is the same. People always want to do this collectively which is also short term and seldom lasts longer than a couple of weeks as most cost money to be part of.

Some diet clubs are very expensive and they all have a monthly subscription fee. So what are you getting? AA does not require a monthly fee if you are in need of support for alcohol dependency. So why should you have to pay money for food dependency? One wonders why there is not a FF (Food Feeders) or FA (Food Abusers).

So if you are required to pay a monthly fee, then it is immediately a business and it is again commercially geared to take cash off a desperate person who is in need of help to create wealth somewhere else for someone else. In my opinion that is bad enough but some of these clubs who are internationally renowned not only charge you a joining fee and a monthly subscription, they also market their "approved" and "clinically approved" products to their own members, encouraging them to purchase their unique brand and release recipes which in each recipe contains at least one of their "unique brand" products.

This is astronomically clever marketing. They gain a base of clientele, they gain a monthly subscription and encourage member recruitment of other members which will give you stars and points which reduces your fees which is a case of loose a little on the swings to gain a lot more on the slides *and* they have a guaranteed secure market for their products which are also very over priced and the quantities are extremely small in comparison to other brands of the same product but belonging to the club, one would never mention the fact that after eating your dinner you are still ravenous. They have weekly meetings where you are weighed in, on a named and shamed basis so loose weight you will as no one wants to be humiliated in front of 30 or 40 other people who are all standing behind the same door, "tut tutting" at your lack of weight loss. Then there is the annual prise giving for the one fatty that lost the most weight. No pressure at all.

There are hundreds of websites on the net which offer up recipes with a shopping list. Well they are very nice and the food look wonderful however, I am a working average person, I cannot afford salmon and snoek, halibut and taco shells. Asparagus and lemon grass are treats not daily events. I travel around, where in the world could I store a frozen low calorie sugar free yoghurt which is the snack item. Apple would be more my speed actually. If you have a family, the cost of the foods in those recipes will not be sustainable. Realism is important. If it is real it will work. Money does matter and while those iffy foods will be nice for a week, like a holiday, I have to come home to reality at some point, we all do.

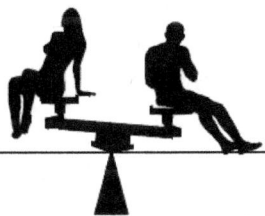

Food and Body Analysis Clinics

These are the scientific approach to weight loss people.

There are many schools of thought in regard to eat butter, bad butter, drink milk, milk is bad…. There are many opinions but analysis clinics take the cake on all argument.

Some take blood, some take urine samples. You pay – a lot. R4500.00 sign on fee and a monthly membership which includes free future analysis, a cardboard fold up menu guide and weekly meetings.

You are issued a lifestyle analysis questionnaire. Well you know, your grandpa could tell you that a sedentary (little activity) lifestyle with bacon and egg breakfast, burger lunch and pizza dinner would make you fat and you should not consume so much fat and oils, hidden sodium(salt) and exercise and he, bless him, did not even have a machine or computer and he also would not have taken your salary away from you to tell you this.

They seem to have different stories for everyone. Some people have been told they should never, ever have touched a carbohydrate (pumpkin, potatoes, rice, bread) and it is due to that mere and one fact that they are overweight. Well here is the news, when you were born the instruction manual clearly was not issued. How in the world would your mom have known that?

One woman told me she was told by *the computer* that she was highly allergic to onions and garlic. It was the downfall of her life according to *the computer*. I stood in amazement; she was absolutely sold on this idea. Now I had known this woman for a couple of months. Our kids were in the same school. I had run into her several times in the same mall I shopped in and I had personally seen her throwing the large strawberry milkshakes with the fresh cream and sprinkles down her throat with her rather large daughter following suit but it was defiantly the onions in her head. So who was I to disagree with a state of the art analysis computer?

The pharmacy assistant, a young man in his 30's who was of very slim build was told he should never eat broccoli or cabbage, literally poison for him. Odd that he had eaten it his whole life and had not succumbed to any ills but that was the reason he never put on any real weight. Not that he had a fast metabolism, the man never walked he ran. He never stood still, he was a nervous wreck and fussed over unseen and invisible dust on the counter. But it was the broccoli's fault. The computer said so.

I have not met anyone who stayed the course, ate the diet prescribed by the computer and lost weight, in fact I just have never met anyone at all who stayed the course period. All payments are upfront. Many people buy into these weird and wonderful ideas. Millions are spent year in and year out. There is no season for weight loss. Advertisers still pull the "get slim for summer" but summer is different in different countries so it is a fluid and moving market. Simple breakfast cereals pull that old rabbit out of the hat every summer.

The gorgeously beautiful sexy sun kissed 19 year old in the red bikini rubbing her French manicured tanned hand over a non existent bulge of stomach giving you the six week challenge. Really? Are you really going to believe that you are going to look like her by eating breakfast cereal for six weeks and which cereal box tastes better than product? Yet stand in that isle and watch over a month end period how many middle aged woman buy it and it has always made me smile, how people are psychologically impacted by marketing. They reach up with one hand and the other automatically touches the stomach as the mind is so dented with the idea of the flat stomach through constant marketing, it has now become a fact in his or her head. This cereal will reduce your stomach. Yes, it will IF you have constipation issues, which you should not have if you just drank sufficient water per day anyway and you are probably too young to be internalizing and thinking about your bowel anyway. You will get to that point when you are old and bran is the highlight of the day but not now. And that cereal is expensive too. Shoppers are interesting, watch woman in the shampoo isle, they constantly touch their hair.

Woman in the sweets isle, they covertly look around them before snapping up a chocolate and pushing it under something else in the basket. Look into peoples baskets and trolleys, they never display the sweets on the top of the other items. Sweets are also at the cashiers and people do the "grab" as a last minute thing, like an after thought and rush them guiltily through with other things. People are amazingly fascinating. If you are in a hurry to get around the store, the sweets isle is the best access route, it is almost always devoid of traffic.

It is really what you want to believe and what you convince yourself of that makes the choices for you. Decisions are different as in order to make a decision, you need some education behind it.

A lot of people are quiet content with what they are, how they look and whatever size they are but they are perpetually on the hunt for the perfect diet, just to be seen to be doing something about what they think others don't approve of, their weight. To some it is a form of attention seeking, to others it is company and friendship and 99.9% of people want to part of something that is bigger than themselves. Something overwhelming and impossible to understand, command, gain control of, and exactly why the diet industry is so massive. The 3 major world industries relative to woman are diet, cosmetics and religion.

Dieting is like Dating. Exciting to begin with, then comes the part where you have to motivate yourself, then the boredom, then you are forcing it, then your friends are encouraging it, then you slip, then you are in self recrimination, then the break up and then the guilt, to start it all over again. The highs and the lows but each time your body does not bounce back as fast as your emotions did when you dated. Your body is hurting, feasting, fasting and registering signals of store now, balloon now, save yourself....and those jeans you hoped would fit are further and further removed from sight and reach.

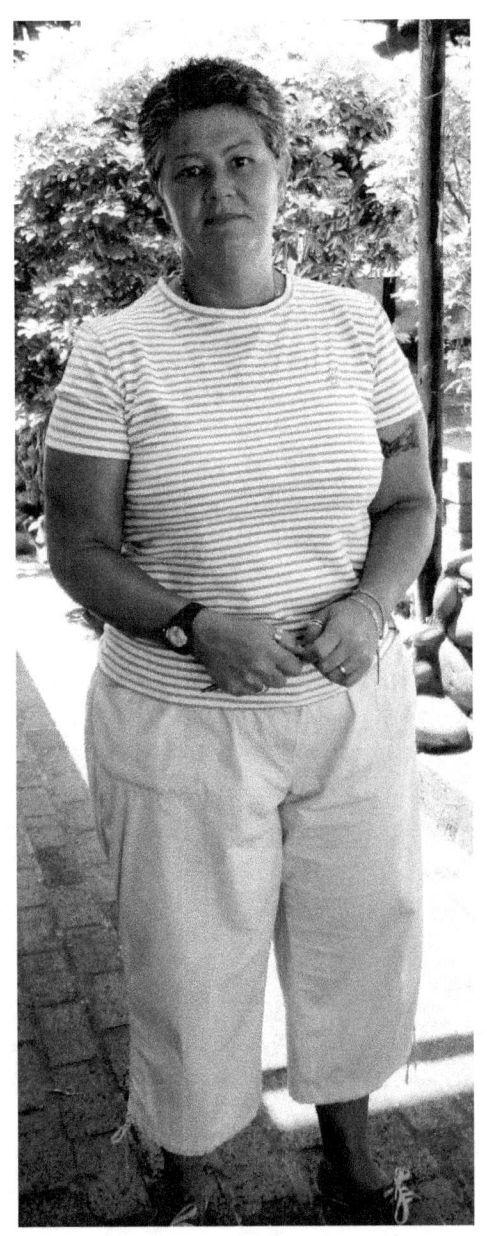

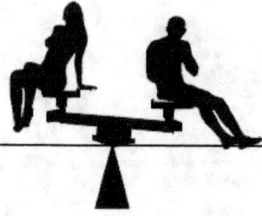

Self Sabotage

Self Sabotage is actually a gene. A great many people are born with it and it is in this gene that when things are going well people change the formula and it all goes south. People born without this gene are generally successful and they are in control of their lives, their relationships, their finances and their futures.

When you are losing weight and it is going well for you, it may not be as fast as we would like but then we now live in a microwave society, you did not put the weight on in 3 weeks but the weight loss package says lose 15kg in 3 weeks and there stands busty babe with a before and after having lost nothing but a few minutes of time in a photo shoot and you chose to believe it. If you are healthy, you feel you have more energy, you lose slowly and your body is adjusting to its new size and shape and you do not have pockets of skin forming you are on a winning track here. Don't change what is a winner for you.

Don't sabotage yourself no matter what marketing you are exposed to or what advice your friends give you. This is all about you and you learning to be you all over again and to be comfortable with yourself.

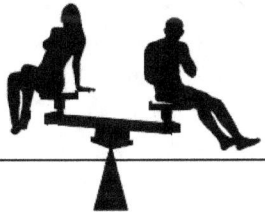

Binge eaters

I had a friend, her name was Pat but behind her back people called her Fat. She was a very very large person and she seldom ate much at all in front of anyone. She was successful in her job, a high powered insurance agent, worked corporate accounts. In this position came the perks of entertainment allowances, large entertainment allowances, the kind that romances the client to sign on the line. It was expected for her to wine and dine her corporate clients and partners and their attorneys and whoever it took to charm into the deal. Many steaks and glasses of alcohol later, Pat went from medium build to fat, to obese, to clinically obese to chronically obese.

She tried various pills, then clubs, then shakes, laxatives, drops and failed in all. When we had social braais at her home as she always insisted we entertained in her home, bring and braai nights and a beautiful home it was, the men would braai the meat as men do, the woman would chat on the patio as woman do and because there were always so many people the meat was placed into the oven pans and left warming while the rest was on the grill.

On one occasion, the two general bathrooms were busy as the kids had been swimming and I had to use her personal bathroom off her bedroom. As I passed her cupboard I could not help noticing that an entire oven pan full of various cuts of meat was sitting sizzling on the shelf of her underwear. I just could not help myself. I opened the door. There were bites taken out of the meat and thrown back into the pan, borewors, steaks, lamb chops and ribs, all had bites taken out. It was like an animal had gotten hold of the pan. I put it back exactly as I found it. I watched her throughout the evening, decanting meat from one pan to another plate, running around the patio offering from the plate in hand, this way no one would ever know a huge heap of meat went missing.

She often excused herself to go to the bathroom, but always pushed her bedroom door on, and when she came out always wiping her mouth with the back of her hand. I made it my mission to go use her bathroom again and checked on the pan of meat, it was eaten down to the bones lying in a little sauce. She had successfully eaten an entire pan of meat on her own, enough for 6 adults easily.

Unfortunately over time her jolly cheer wore thin on the client base as she grew fatter and her usefulness had waned in the company and she was retrenched. The truth was, her own clients now found her vulgar and offensive to be with, an embarrassment. There were thinner, more attractive agents to have fun with at lunch time.

Pat was retrenched with a very healthy package, but her mental illness with food had become such that she feared not having enough. She would call each of her friends in turn begging food and groceries.

We all fell for it at first and would take her boot loads not knowing there were several boot loads that had come before and some were still en route until one friend bought her meat and there was a power failure but being on a old small holding there was power to an outbuilding through a generator. This person had the domestic cleaner open the storeroom up and a world of revelation, it looked like a supermarket. Everything was in abundance including meat.

Pat had successfully conned her friends out of food for some months collecting it in her stores under lock and key with large chest freezers containing meat, chicken and fish. It was annoying at first but more than that it was terribly sad. None of us realised just how far her illness with food had gone.

Due to her size, her lack of self confidence and all her issues collectively, she became hostile, personal and abusive to her closest friends. Alcohol became her second dependency and food she ate openly now and the last I heard she had lost the small holding she once so proudly entertained on and was living with friends but was in poor heart health, she had never lost her weight, abused alcohol and her health. I lost touch with her totally after I moved to another province.

Food cannot compensate for self worth.

Food cannot replace your self respect.

Food cannot nullify emotions.

Food cannot keep you company.

Food is not a whip to hurt yourself with

Food is fuel, tasty, interesting and colourful but it is just fuel for our bodies to function.

Food can heal us, but too little of it or too much of it can and will harm us.

Develop a good relationship with food.

It is there, it is accessible. It is also expensive and needs appreciation.

Use it in it's best possible forms to optimise your body and your general health.

Take the time and present it properly even if you eat alone.

Set your table, use the table mat and the knife and fork, use the napkin and set a glass for what you are drinking. Bring the cold water to the table. Treat yourself worthy of a meal. Your table is your restaurant. You are your waiter. Food is the reward.

Celebrities have also had issues with weight. Rich, powerful people we admire for achievement but when you read the battles they have fought we can relate and look into their lives with sympathy.

OPRAH'S BINGE EATING YEARS

In previous years, Oprah Winfrey's very public struggle with her weight has seen her slim down to a svelte figure, only to gain it all back again. She's also tried various dieting techniques, such as eating only vegan food for a short period of time, and going on a detox diet that eliminated caffeine, alcohol, meat, and sugar, among other things.

These weight loss diets are all well and good, but it wasn't until Oprah was able to acknowledge her feelings toward food that she could move forward with healthier food strategies. She realised she was using food as an emotional crutch. Once, she famously ate 30 pounds of macaroni and cheese after her artistic endeavors received poor ratings. Oprah herself stated that she has "abuse(d) food" by binge eating.

Binge eating brings about more complications than just weight gain; it also raises the risk of insomnia, high cholesterol, and menstrual problems. Binge eaters are more likely to suffer from diabetes, gallbladder disease, and decreased mobility. This type of food disorder is often linked to emotional eating, and it is also associated with other mental disorders like depression.

Focus on healthy food choices

After Oprah changed her perceptions about food and became aware of her emotional eating, she began to focus on healthy food choices.

Her special daily diet focuses on foods that are flavorful and filling; the complex carbohydrates help her stay full all day, and make her less likely to binge eat.

Oprah has also struggled with exercise. Around the time that she changed her perceptions toward eating, she began to work out five to six days per week, for about an hour each day. She began slowly, with walking, and ramped up the cardio as she began to get fit again. Strength training is also essential because it helps prevent age-related muscle loss.

Many binge eaters live a life of secrecy and shame but according to international research binge eating is more common than anorexia or bulimia.

When she came under fire for a bad show and movie all these stories were coming out and about letting the Oprah backlash begin. She handled the stress by asking her chef to make her macaroni and cheese and bread pudding. "I ate about 30 pounds worth. I'm not kidding I really, literally, went into a tailspin with it."

Winfrey's not alone in using food to fight emotional distress. A 2007 study by Harvard Medical School psychiatrists found binge eating disorder is more common than either anorexia or bulimia, affecting 3.5% of women and 2% of men.

Binge eaters don't just eat too much dessert at their favourite restaurant or pig out at a party. Binge eaters often eat huge amounts -- entire large pizzas and cartons of ice cream, for example -- and overeat at least once a week for three months, according to experts. They often eat alone because they're embarrassed over how much they're eating, and then feel disgusted with themselves and guilty afterward.

What fuels the binges is a desire to get away from an unpleasant feeling you're eating because you want something inside of you to numb out. Many binge eaters say they've managed to stop by using self-help techniques.

Advice on what to do if you're a binge eater

1. **Realise you can change**

   The most pervasive misconception about binge eating is that it's hopeless,

2. *Identify your emotional distress*

Oprah says at first, she thought it was all about the food. "I thought I just wanted some macaroni." It took her a while to connect the eating with her emotional distress. "I didn't connect the powerlessness," she said.

3. *Just before a binge, remind yourself why you're binging*

Let's dissect a binge. Before the actual eating occurs, the binger has "food thought" -- a thought that eating would be a good idea.

Before that thought turns into action, try to figure out why you're eating.

4. *Figure out if you're distorting the truth*

Once you identify the emotion that's leading to the binge, you should then ask yourself whether you're upset over nothing.

5. *Feel the sadness*

When something is truly sad, sometimes you just have to feel it.

Just like the rest of us, Oprah Winfrey has her dark moments.

Oprah Article by: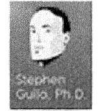

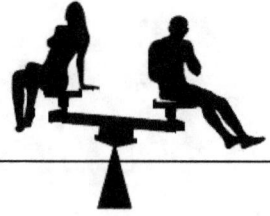

All or Nothing Diets

Only protein

No Carbs

Low Carbs

All vegetarian

Fruitarian

Only Liquids

Sequence Eating

Combination diets

All of the above are highly popular BUT they are not sustainable. You will lose weight in the first week, and you will feel amped that you have energy and you think you are winning the battle. It is like taking a battleship to an argument. Over kill and over done which will put your body into shock and starvation mode. It will register that you are not feeding it adequately so everything you eat will be used up and everything that is not needed will be stored.

Within a couple of weeks you will get bored and you will break it with "ag, I have been so good, this wont hurt." So begins the weight packing again. From that point on, what you have lost you will put back on and more.

You need all the food groups. Each part of our system needs various foods and we need to eat them to survive and to be healthy. We do not need processed food, we do not need extra sugar and we do not need packaged foods or take away or fast food, but you need carbs and fruit and fish and meat and chicken and liquids. You need them all, not one at a time.

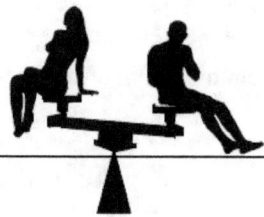

Hair

I have several hairdresser friends and each one has told me the same thing.

They have very few "big girl" clients and when the "big girl" clients do come in their hair is a dying tragedy with over processing, home hack jobs and bad hair fall.

So I started to observe this in large ladies.

Unfortunately this is actually a fact. There was probably one out of 100 I observed that took good care of their hair and 89 of the 100 observations coloured their hair red, plum or black.

I imagine this is the last resort of the range and a cover all evils, shade.

None at all had good cuts and all used ironing tools on their hair making the ends frizz or appear as if a rat had a go at the ends.

At least 50 of the observations had re-growth and scalp visibility.

I do not believe that a colour change is going to change how you feel about yourself in general. You are still going to be discontent, just with a different shade on your head.

A crowning glory tells so much about a woman.

A shiny well maintained head of hair compensates for a great deal.

Your body is already unhealthy, bad health will reflect in your hair and nails as it does with bulimics, anorexics, drug addicts and alcoholics.

A bulimic and anorexic has two tell tale signs that scream the condition.

Enlarged ears (inappropriate size for the scalp). As with aging, the ears and nose grows as cartilage does not stop growing unlike bones. With anorexia and bulimia, the calcium is deficient in the body causing the bone mass to shrink and the cartilage to grow. The body registers natural progression of age in calcium deficiency. Starving it triggers this condition.

The other sign is the hair condition, invariably a painfully thin ponytail as these sufferers will grow their hair to cover the scalp as the gapping is obvious with short cuts.

The lesser obvious sign is gum recession where the teeth should be buried in the gum, there is gapping and almost all people who suffer sensitivity have eating disorders.

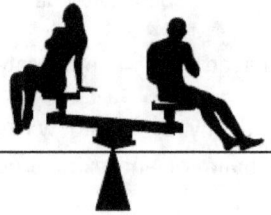

Clothing

More and more people seem to think that wearing really large clothing hides it, it does not. You look like a fridge with a head on it.

Wearing too tight clothing also looks bad. Look in the mirror before you go out. Michelin man comes to mind. If you are overweight, you know it. Dress appropriately. Look good all the time. Large totally groomed people are beautiful. Large people who are not groomed attract ugly names like..."fat chick", "tubby over there"...don't make yourself a target of abuse. Even when you are at home, make it a habit to groom yourself well. Casual is wonderful for weekends, but there is casual and there is slob. Learn to look wonderful in your pyjamas.

A friend of mine was interviewing people for a position in his company. He used agencies but he felt the position needed a very big personality; it was a cold call telesales position. This woman arrived with a big personality and an even bigger body, only she had clothing on that were easily two sizes too small and mostly appropriate for a gym training session.

She was perfect for the job but he did not take her on. He said all the flesh was overwhelming to him and could not see himself working with it all. It was too much. He said she was a mass of face and shine and mammary glands on the desk and it was so "aaaahhhggg!" And he physically shook himself in absolute disgust.

Ladies, men in general are not the stereotype "boob and bums" pigs. Most men are decent human beings. Men may not comment on the frontal flesh expose' for one simple reason, they cannot and would not risk it for fear of being accused of sexual misconduct and harassment, but I assure you they do not like it nor appreciate your generosity of your anatomy display in this area and in the work place.

It took a month to fill the position and it was filled with a very large woman too but she dressed appropriately for the office environment.

When you look great outside you feel great inside and that is what you have been searching for all these years and that feeling is your target. To feel confident, be amazed at your own mobility, be able to use the whole of you, have that energy for life, that enthusiasm you felt was lost and your personality will radiate you.

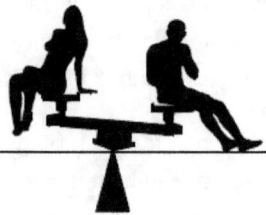

Fat, Finance & Self Esteem

Being overweight has a direct connection to low self esteem, being in financial difficulty and a direct connection to self esteem. Low self esteem and self control are interconnected.

Companies will always overlook the fat person in favour of a thin person for a position as fat has a trail of lack of self control, financial difficulty and low self esteem.

The fat person in the office always has one draw filled with crisps, sweets, snacks and extra cash in case a food vendor happens by. This very person in 99% of the cases has financial woes.

An HR placement agent friend of mine told me that she was having more and more issues with large companies and large corporate companies taking placements of overweight persons. They would be eager to interview on the CV presentation but post interview they were cold on the candidate due to the person being weighted.

Companies look at fat people with tunnel vision, they assume the person is weak willed and open to bribery and fraud, they assume bad health and time the person would be off work, they assume lack of self esteem and they assume financial difficulty. Sadly in most case two out of the three prove correct.

When we cannot manage our weight, we have lost control of ourselves. People who have lost control of themselves do not maintain control over other aspects of their lives either. Their kids are normally spoilt and overweight, their homes are generally not maintained well and their finances are generally not maintained for two reasons. Financial hardship does not mean the person is incapable of making the money or earning it, they just lack the means to control their spend.

I know a person who earned a small fortune every month, I envied her. Single person, no dependants. Her home was lovely, big house, lovely maintained garden, stunning pool and car, the life we all have aspired to at some point or another. But that was from the outside looking in.

The reality of her life was she battled her weight, diet hopping, and was at that point on the Injections. She was a middle average weighted person, for middle age spread. She was also bulimic. Her life was a nightmare. She did not date as she may have had to eat, so she had a lot of first "coffee" dates. She did not get involved as she did not want to get close to anyone, I mean physically close as her breath was acrid all the time and not even the minted gum can disguise that smell. So she was lonely in her lovely home. She had a lot of friends but when you looked at the types she befriended they were users. When she pulled up in her car people did not see her, they looked at her hands and what she was carrying in for them. CD's, gift boxes of chocolates and nuts, perfume, food and all the things that put big smiles on peoples faces. She was popular, and she felt good about her "friends" and they loved having her over, they said. They had missed her.

Sadly she was retrenched. The gifts stopped and so did the invites. No one seemed to miss her anymore.

How many times have you heard people saying about an ex-heavy weight, "they used to be so nice and friendly and always helped others, now they changed since they lost weight."

Did they change or did they just gain self control, self respect and saw through the people that took advantage of their "fat" nature?

When you feel good, look good from your own perspective and you do not need to hear it from others at all, yes it is nice that others recognise your efforts but it is actually about how you feel about yourself that matters the most, you gain something, something extra about yourself, an air of confidence, a grace in your walk, a comfort in your own self and an enlarged capacity of capability. That is when you will see through the falseness of so many things. People, situations, submission, and it is not that she became a "bitch" or he became a "bastard", it is that those who walk the road back to the cross roads that they took the wrong path of weight gain and lost each kilo on the path back to normalcy and health took the hard road as it is not just about losing the weight now, it is about rediscovery and don't fear that path as it is a journey you actually do want to do. It is actually exciting and it is discovery.

When we were younger we were generally bantered and pushed into the lives we have now, we went along with it and something we did not like and other things we just succumbed to as it was easier and we got on. Now you can do it all over again and you will find things that you do not like and things that are just not what you thought they were and maybe even some people are no longer a good fit for you and it is okay. You are on a journey and it is yours and you need to own it.

The financial aspect of overweight people is that they settle. They are used to the fast food, the quick, the easy and the instant. Most will live in mediocre homes with mediocre cars and jobs and that is the lot of the weighted person with floral and stripes and mismatched everything in their homes. Oh there is a sound reason for the bad décor too, food was more important than décor. I have heard a million times, I can't eat a pillow or a throw or a rug. There are very few CEO's of companies that are fat people, there are very few fat success stories. Company owners are invariably too stressed to eat endless plates of food and have far more pressing issues than to think about what's the next meal.

When you have your weight under control you will invariably bring your finances under control as well and where food was a comfort to you before, achievement will replace that and money comes, when you work hard, efficiently and effectively, the money comes.

Food is a pleasure but it can be a poison as Heroin is a drug and a poison, used in pharmaceuticals correctly it is a medicine.

Every single thing in life has up and down sides. Make the best of everything that goes into your body. Use your body like you would your best suit. It is after all the suit your soul is in for now.

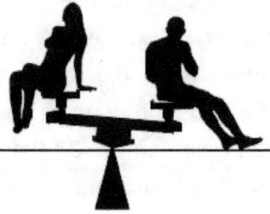

End IT

How many diets have you started, fell of and felt like a failure? Why set yourself up for a fall all the time. All of it, the concepts, the diets, the expenses, they are doing way more damage than you would believe. Not only to your body, but to your mental and emotional state. It will impact everything in your life eventually. You interpersonal relationships, your self confidence and your self esteem. You will feel worthless eventually, you will feel like the ultimate failure and you will eventually look the part BUT you are not a failure.

You are just going about winning in the incorrect method.

There are two ways to play any game ...play not to loose or play to win.

Both ways you get to stay in the game but one will make you feel like you are carrying a ton of lead on your back and the other will see wings under your feet.

Personally, I have wings, I am a winner. I play every aspect of my life to win.

Set your goal, identify your obstacles and evaluate which route around, over or under then but let nothing and no persons stand in your way. It is not about the past, it is not how you looked and how you felt way back when. It is about now and the future.

We can do nothing to change yesterday. The burger was eaten, the milkshake is sitting in memory on the lips and the chips on the hips.

How we felt way back then, the memories of how happy we were when we were slim and trim actually had nothing to do with our shape then. It all has to do with being in control.

When we were in our early adulthood we had support we did not even identify. In some cases resented. Our parents were guarding us from a distance, our teachers wanted us to succeed, neighbours kept an eye out, every adult was responsible for every child in the street, it was a different place and world and we were in control because of the "invisible" support we had.

We had just so much money and it was an easier life, bought the bus ticket, made your sandwich for work lunch, had only three outfits and rotation was just fine as were the 3 pairs of shoes we owned and borrowing clothing and swapping was a way of life. We managed, we always came through and life was simple.

The world changed and it all seems so out of control now. We never know if we will have enough to get through the month, we never know what the day will bring and how much the next crisis will cost us, it is so quick and so easy to lose everything now. Life became complicated and we have less and less time to concentrate on us. We all choices and they worked out but today you have to minimize choices and consciously make decisions because there seems so little time to go back and do over. Life moves too fast now.

End IT, stop making choices and start making decisions. Realise the difference between the two. A choice is when someone phones you and says you qualified for another phone, you can have ABC or CBA. You fear you may not qualify again and yours is showing a little wear. You make a choice. You take a deal. You did not need another contract or expense and it is not the phone that you ideally wanted. If you just saved a little you would have had what you really wanted a little later and you would really have liked and appreciate it . **Now you settled**....again and it is so bland. It is so disappointing that after you unpacked the phone, it is so disinteresting you actually start looking at the packaging, really? Well the cardboard is just about how you are feeling about the phone. This was an emotive purchase. You felt acknowledged when they called and you felt important for that period. Now you have buyers remorse. It was not the instrument, it was the emotion you felt while you were finalising the deal. You were good enough. THEY wanted YOUR business. No. They wanted your money. You were a sucker.

Your diet is the same. **Don't settle. Never settle.** Know what you want to eat. Decide and list your items before you enter a store. Do not shop randomly. It is expensive to do so and you will be tempted to buy things you have an appetite for rather than what you need. If you find you do not have the discipline to shop on a list, do online shopping. Online shopping is a sobering experience if you are trying to diet and have a budget. The shopping cart runs your total as you spend. No surprises. No miscalculations. No over purchases.

If store A does not have what you want, never take a substitute. Never be lazy when it comes to you. You count. You have one life and it is so important, special. Go to the next store and put into your body what you intended.

If you ran out of mascara would you make a dash into the garage and grab the black paint, if you ran out of powder puff would you borrow the roller? Well why not? You are doing it for the inside of your body, why should you not follow through for the outside? Because people can see it....so what makes you think that they cannot see the kilo's packing onto your butt and hips?

Remember that people are more inclined to make a nasty comment than a kind one. You can stand with all the smiles in the world but when you turn your back eyebrows raise and someone is going to say something and not something kind either.

Be in control and that is what is essentially missing from your life right now and each time you purchase another diet remedy you are digging away at the foundation under you but keep it real. Hang closely and tightly to reality.

It has always fascinated me how quickly a woman will react to a man having an unzipped fly and they actually act self righteous as if the poor bloke is deliberate in an attempt to offend them in particular when in 100% of cases it was a total oversight but woman have no problem in hanging the mammaries half out, pushed up under the jowls or squashed into over tight clothing leaving nothing to anyone's imagination and over and above have this wheel of wall to wall flesh tubing around their backs. Not nice and not pleasant to work with for other females or males. Look at yourself in the mirror.

Averted eyes are not accepting eyes. Your colleagues should be able to look you in the face, in the eyes with openness. Not address the cabinet when talking to you. No matter how big you are, there is appropriate clothing as sizes to fit you.

Too tight clothing does not make you look younger. Because someone else is doing it does not make it right. Fat legs do not look good in short skirts. Fat woman should not wear shorts.

Do not compete with your daughters, no matter how they tell you to be "cool" and "with it", there is decorum. Dignity is essential to successful ageing.

Self control will bring you self respect and self respect brings with it a whole new world including not allowing yourself to continue abusing yourself. Never confuse self respect with being egotistical and self righteous either.

Reformed and reborn anything and anyone is generally irritating to others. Have you ever had the misfortune to sit in the company of an ex smoker. Some ex over eaters tend to become self righteous too. Enjoy your new self and bring happiness and pleasure. I have heard on a number of occasions people remarking "she was such a nice person when she was fat, now she is nasty." I have also heard "fat people are jolly", not really, they are unhappy inside but compensate with the girl /boy / woman / man who will always baby sit, feed the cats, stay late at work, clean up after the office party.

Don't be a mat either. Value yourself. Others already do.

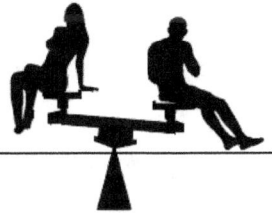

Programme & Book

The calorie counter is included in the book however should you wish to access the online programme email susan@writersink.co.za to open your access to the online version of the counter. It makes your life that much easier as it is a self calculating version and takes all the hard work away from you.

You will receive a link via email where you will have access to the diet program from any computer in the world including your cell phone (smart phone).

Enter your own password and you will access your program

Ideally when a woman is reducing weight, the maximum calories she should eat is 1200- 1600 per day.

Ideally when a man is reducing weight, the maximum calories he should eat is 1600 - 2000 per day.

In this plan set all the portion values to 0. Scroll the list and see what you would LIKE to eat for the day. Check the portions of that food to 1 in the portion column. At the bottom of the counter you would have automatically totalled your calories. Adjust them according to a breakfast meal, a snack, lunch, a snack and supper and a snack.

Explore the sheet, click on the speech bubbles for idea and opinions, hints and tips.

Click on the clips for recipes.

The programme is interactive, as an update or change is made by our programmers or another member the sheet will update, if a change is made by you, the sheet will update for others to see.

Below is an example of a +-1200 calorie day plan

Breakfast
Two slices of toast – buttered lightly
Boiled egg
Tea /coffee with milk

Snack
Apple

Lunch
2 slices white bread sandwich of cheese tomato and lettuce and cucumber

Snack
½ cup sliced biltong or 2 cups popcorn

Dinner
Roasted Chicken breast
½ cup cooked carrots
½ cup broccoli
Medium steamed or baked potato

The above is calculated to 1214 calories, there is room for a blob of butter on the dinner potato, or some gravy, an added salad or a baked apple or roasted banana for desert.

A cup of milk is calculated into the above allowing for milk in tea or coffee. Sweeteners are a choice. I have not found that 2 teaspoons of sugar have done any damage if you only drink 3 cups of tea or coffee per day. If you have excessive sugar per cup, you need to look at how you wish to handle that.

This plan is all about flexibility. Some days I did not feel like meat and chose only vegetable and salads and some days I only wanted meat or snacked out on popcorn and biltong to replace supper entirely as it was a Saturday and I was camping out in front of the TV. I stayed on the 1400 count per day to begin with. Within 2 weeks I could feel my metabolism kicking in. You need your metabolism to burn the fuel you put into the body. Too slow a metabolism and you store food. It parks and the only way to kick up your metabolism is to eat correctly. Don't think by starving your body it will burn more, it actually slows down. Your body gets used to 1400 count and then you drop by 100 to 1300 and continue for another two weeks and see how you feel. Listen to your body. Don't drop below 1200 calories per day. There is no need, you will just set yourself up for a fall again. Some days you don't really want to eat it all so have something smaller of higher calorie count. Other days you may feel you want more quantity so have lots with lower counts.

If you are way above your weight level, the way to calculate your needs are as follows:
Calculate your kilo weight to pounds.
Kilo weight x 2.2 – weight in pounds.
Weight in pounds x 12 = ( ) and subtract 1000
If answer is less than 1200 stay on 1200

Use a combination of vegetables to make soups and stews. Shuffle and change to suit yourself and your family needs. If you are putting the entire family on your plan you calculate for one and cook for three or four and serve accordingly, just allow a bit more for the men in the house.

In the speech bubble on the left hand side of the sheet, you will find attached recipes. In the attachment clip you will find ideas and pics and suggestions.

Feel free to add your own by clicking on the clip block and upload your own recipes, ideas.

You can set alarms and reminders in the bell icon for yourself, the program will send you a reminder email of your reminder.

Feel free to be interactive with other users. This is yours. Make the best of it.

You are controlling your diet, your intake, your health and your life. New features will constantly update on the programme.

Food Type	Quantity	Protein grams	Carbs grams	Fat grams	Total Calories
Meat & Poultry Proteins					
Roasted Skinless Chicken thigh	1 Cup	36	0	15	293
Roasted chicken breast	1 Cup	43	0	5	268
Roasted skinless chicken drumstick	1 Cup	40	0	8	241
Roasted Chicken wing	Per single	6	0	2	43
Beef Sirloin	Palm size	50	0	26	225
Beef Brisket Braised	Palm size or 3 slices	46	0	34	247
Mince pan browned/cooked	1/2 cup	44	0	10	139
Meatball medium	1	6	4	5	85
Salmon Steak 200 grams	200g	44	0	7	155
Canned Pink Salmon 140g	140g	17	0	5	118
Pork Chop medium	1 chop	36	0	18	314
Tuna Steak	200g	50	0	5	156
Canned Tuna in Water	140g	20	0	6	109
Haddock Steak	200g	42	0	1	95
Shrimp	200g	18	0	1	84
Crab	200g	16	0	1	82
Eggs And Dairy					
3 Egg Omelette	3	18	0	13	189
1 large egg	1	6	0	5	65
1 large egg fried	1	6	0	7	87
Scrambled eggs 3	3	18	0	13	189
Whole milk	1 cup	8	11	8	146
2% milk	1 cup	8	11	5	102
Cottage Cheese	1/2 cup	13	4	5	110
Cottage Cheese low fat	1/2 cup	14	3	1	81
Plain Yoghurt 125ml	125ml	9	11	8	149
Plain Greek Yoghurt 125	125ml	13	17	4	154

Food Type	Quantity	Protein grams	Carbs grams	Fat grams	Total Calories
Carbohydrates (Non Starchy Veg)					
Apple Medium	1	0	19	0	64
Asparagus	1 cup	2	4	2	12
Avocado	1	3	13	21	213
Banana	1	1	27	3	101
Blueberries	1 cup	1	18	0	63
Broccoli	1 cup	3	6	0	27
Cabbage shredded	1 cup	1	4	0	3
Carrots medium	1 cup	1	6	0	18
Cauliflower	1 cup	2	5	0	19
Cherries 1	1 cup	1	19	0	70
Cucumber slices	1 cup	0	2	0	2
Fresh onions chopped	1 cup	2	16	0	4
Grapefruit pink	1 med	1	29	0	54
Grapes	1 cup	1	29	0	114
Green Beans 1	1 cup	4	9	0	32
Kiwi Fruit	1 unit	1	13	3	46
Garlic fresh	per Pod	1	4	0	4
Melon cubed	1 cup	1	16	0	62
Nectarine	1 unit	1	14	0	54
Orange	1 unit	2	22	0	75
Peach large	1unit	1	9	0	35
Plum	1 plum	1	8	0	28
Pumpkin	1 cup	2	7	0	38
Rasberries	1 cup	2	16	0	40
Spinach boiled or steamed	1 cup	5	7	0	31
Spinach Fresh	1 cup	1	1	0	6
Squash medium	1 unit	2	6	0	22
Strawberries	1 cup	1	11	0	36
Tomato medium	1 unit	1	2	0	6
Watermelon diced	1 cup	1	12	1	47

Food Type	Quantity	Protein grams	Carbs grams	Fat grams	Total Calories
Oils For cooking & Salad dressings					
Olive Oil	1 Tbls	0	0	14	126
Coconut Oil	1 Tbls	0	0	14	126
Avocado Oil	1 Tbls	0	0	14	126

Food Type	Quantity	Protein grams	Carbs grams	Fat grams	Total Calories
Fats (Nuts & Seeds)					
Almonds	1/4 cup	6	2	19	163
Hazels	1/4 cup	4	5	18	188
Walnuts	1/4 cup	4	4	20	205
Pecans	1/4 cup	3	4	20	195
Macadamia	1/4 cup	2	4	3	209

Food Type	Quantity	Protein grams	Carbs grams	Fat grams	Total Calories
Miscellaneous					
Apple Juice	125ml	0	27	0	108
Apple Sauce	1 cup	0	28	0	99
Bacon pan fried	1 strip	3	0	4	45
Biltong salted	1/4 cup	12	6	1	81
Butter	1 Tbls	0	0	12	104
Bovril	1 tsp	28	8	0	80
Coffee black	1 cup	0	0	0	0
Couscous cooked	1/2 cup	3	18	0	88
Feta Cheese	1 x 10cm	4	1	6	75
Grape Juice	1 cup	0	31	0	124
Lobster cooked	1 unit	23	2	1	105
Orange Juice	1 cup	2	25	0	102
Peanut Butter	2 Tbls	4	3	8	97

Food Type	Quantity	Protein grams	Carbs grams	Fat grams	Total Calories
Miscellaneous cont.../					
Pineapple Chunks	1 cup	1	20	2	78
Popcorn	1 cup	1	6	1	24
Potato	medium	6	48	0	105
Raisins	1/2 cup	1	23	1	90
Rice White cooked	1 cup	9	89	2	206
Rice Brown cooked	1 cup	10	83	7	215
Sweet Potato Baked in skin	1 unit	4	37	6	144
Tea Black	1 cup	0	0	0	0
White bread	1 slice	12	8	8	64
Tomato Sauce	1/2 cup	2	4	0	18
White rolls per	1 unit	18	14	9	96
Soy Sauce	1/2 cup	2	0	0	8
Brown bread per slice	1 slice	9	9	11	84
Cheese Rolls per	1 unit	64	38	64	204
Provita per	1 unit	8	16	2	66

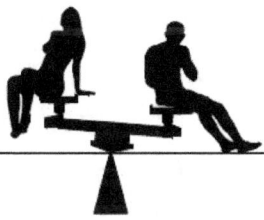

Authors Note:

I learnt the hardest possible way,
that if it is to be it is up to me.

I know how horrid it is to be fat, it is a
nasty word I know and not politically or
socially correct any longer, we are
supposed to say, big bodied, large person,
weighted or challenged but the facts
remain, it is fat, it is rolls of ugly tissue
we squash into clothing, hide under
clothing or just give up and let it all hang
out.

Whether you want to be politically correct or incorrect, fat is ruining everything in your life, it is taking away a large percentage of who you really are, it minimises the real you who is locked inside the mass and YOU alone can change it all. You can make a choice to remain in your prison of fat or you can make a decision to break out.

Enjoy and feel free to communicate with me through the publishers at Writersink.co.za

Health is your primary Wealth.

Sitting is the new smoking.

Chris Gillam

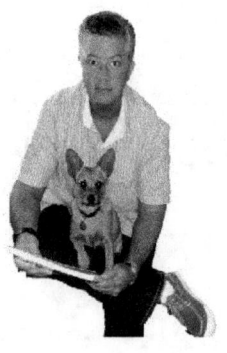

www.ingramcontent.com/pod-product-compliance
Lightning Source LLC
Chambersburg PA
CBHW060644290526
45793CB00001B/384